S0-AHQ-383

Table of Contents

INTRODUCTION

If you're someone who is dealing with diabetes, there's no question that you must be paying attention to what you eat each day. The foods you put into your body are going to have a very strong influence on not only how well you feel, but on how well you handle this condition altogether.

By making smart food choices, you can maintain control over your diabetes and live the lifestyle that you want to lead.

The following 101 foods will do just that. We've selected the top picks that you should include in your diet plan regularly so you no longer have to wonder what to eat.

This list is meant to encourage you to broaden your eating choices. This prevents the boredom that many experience by getting stuck on limited diets, and often leads to "cheating" which can have very unhealthy consequences.

Some diabetics can eat all of these foods, but that doesn't mean all diabetics can eat all of these foods. Even though these are all healthy foods, your body is the final judge of which of these foods are best for YOU. So listen to your body! If a particular meal spikes your sugar, isolate the food that caused it and eliminate it from future choices while looking for something that will give you a similar food taste and experience.

These foods are very rich in nutrients and will help you maintain steady blood sugar levels throughout the day. If you eat a wide variety of them on a regular basis throughout the week, you'll be feeding your body right and energizing yourself for all the different activities that you choose to pursue.

So let's get started and show you the top 101 foods that are best for diabetics.

Attention All Eagle Eyes: We've had a number of people proof this book before we released it to you, but there is a chance you might spot something that was missed. If you find a typo or other obvious error please send it to us. And if you're the first one to report it, we'll send you a free gift! Send to: millwoodmedia@gmail.com

GET THE LATEST DIABETES RESEARCH
AND CLINICALLY PROVEN METHODS
THAT THE BIG PHARMACEUTICAL
COMPANIES DON'T WANT YOU TO KNOW
TO CURE YOUR DIABETES NATURALLY.

DiabeticDoctor.com

DIABETES DIET

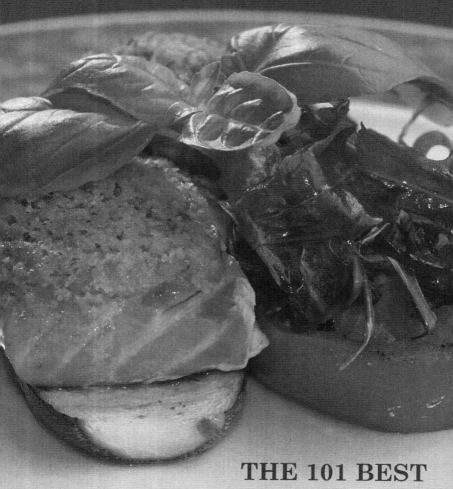

THE 101 BEST
DIABETIC FOODS

ALMONDS

Almonds are a healthy fat-rich food that you should be including in your diet plan. They're rich in manganese and vitamin E, along with being a great source of phosphorus. Adding almonds to your meal can help to decrease the spike in blood sugar that's experienced when carbohydrates are consumed, making them especially attractive for those with diabetes. One study in the American Society for Nutrition found that when almonds were added to a carbohydrate-based meal, they helped to lower the level of insulin release that was necessary to maintain blood glucose levels in a healthy range.

The many benefits of almonds can be enjoyed in more ways than just eating the seed (no, it's technically not a "nut" as most people presume). Almond butter is tasty and more nutritious than peanut butter. Almond milk is a healthy alternative to cow's milk or soy milk. Though much lower in protein, it also has fewer calories and has a smaller impact on blood sugar. Almond flour is highly nutritious, easy to use, gluten-free and great for baking. It's also high in protein, low in carbohydrates and low in sugars, making it a great low-glycemic alternative to regular flours.

APPLES

If you're looking for a sweet treat to calm your cravings, consider an apple. Apples are a natural source of healthy sugar for the body and due to their higher fiber content, won't spike the blood sugar level nearly as much as other sugars. Apples also contain phytonutrients, which play a large role in regulating blood sugar levels, so again are of great benefit to those who have diabetes. A study published in the Gastroenterology Journal also noted that those who consumed apple pectin showed a delayed gastric-emptying time compared to those eating other fiber based foods. At only 81 calories per medium apple, they're easy to add into your diet plan and will put a stop to hunger between your meals.

Pair them together with a small dose of almond or peanut butter for healthy fats and protein and you'll have a very well balanced snack.

APRICOTS

Another great fruit to consider adding to your day is apricots. This fruit is well known for it's vitamin A content, which is a very strong antioxidant that can help to protect you against free radical damage. In addition to this, apricots are an excellent source of fiber with can help to keep you regular with your bowel movements and help to control blood sugar levels.

As an added benefit, apricots are high in beta-carotene as well, which can help ward off heart disease. Go for this sweet treat containing a measly 16 calories per fruit any time in the day.

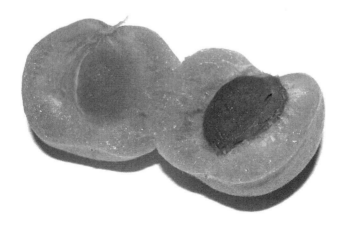

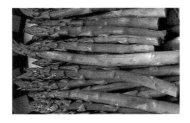

ASPARAGUS

One vegetable that's jam packed with nutrients that you'll definitely want to consider adding to your diet is asparagus. This food only has 43 calories per serving and boasts over 100% of your total daily vitamin K needs. It's also a rich source of folate, vitamin C, vitamin A, tryptophan, thiamine, and riboflavin. In addition to this, asparagus will provide strong anti-inflammatory benefits in the body along with antioxidant protection, which can help to reduce the issues associated with Type 2 diabetes. Coming in with over 3 grams of dietary fiber per serving, they are also going to help to lower your risk of blood sugar spikes and crashes following a meal.

AVOCADOS

One food that's excellent for the diabetic as it's a great source of healthy fats that will help to keep blood sugar levels stable after eating a mixed meal with proteins and carbohydrates is the avocado. This food is rich in essential fatty acids, which will help to protect against heart disease and provide anti-inflammatory benefits. Avocados are also loaded in vitamin K and dietary fiber, which is important for keeping your heart healthy and blood clotting properly. This food contains less than two grams of sugar per cup serving and is also ranked low on the glycemic index scale. Add it to salads, on top of sandwiches, or mix it into a dip to serve alongside your favorite raw veggies.

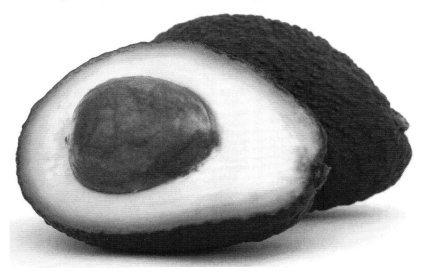

BANANAS

Bananas are a fruit that some diabetics fear as they do tend to be higher in carbohydrates than other fruits, but there are many benefits to including these in your diet that you should consider. First, bananas are very rich in pro-vitamin A, which can help to protect against health problems such as cancer, cardiovascular disease, as well as diabetes. In addition to this, bananas are a very rich source of potassium, which is a nutrient that's very beneficial for helping to lower blood pressure and promote strong bones.

With their high fiber content, as long as you pair these with a source of protein or healthy fat, they should be fine for you to eat. Choose a smaller sized banana if you're worried about the carbohydrate count and you'll easily reap all the benefits this fruit has to offer.

BARLEY

A food that is extremely high in dietary fiber, barley is a great complex carb to add to your diet. Often those with diabetes tend to fear foods higher in carbohydrates, but if you choose properly they can be added. Barley is slow digesting and the fiber found will help to slow the passage of food through the body, helping to regulate blood sugar nicely. Researchers noted that when subjects in a study were given two test meals, one with barley and the other without, the meal containing the barley showed a blunted insulin response compared to the meal without. Barley is also very high in niacin, which can help to protect against cardiovascular disease as well.

BASIL

Basil is one spice that you might want to consider adding to your diet plan to help boost the anti-inflammatory benefits you receive. This spice has a eugenol component that helps to provide relief of the symptoms associated with inflammatory conditions including diabetes.

BEEF, LEAN

Very lean beef tenderloin is a great protein choice for those who have diabetes as it provides a great protein source and will also supply you with the iron that's critical for red blood cell production. Lean beef is also very rich in vitamin B12 and vitamin B6, which are two vitamins that help ward off cardiovascular disease. Finally, beef is also rich in zinc content, which will help to promote a strong immune system and prevent the onset of illness.

BEETS

One often overlooked vegetable that many people forget about that you should consider re-introducing into your diet is the beet. Beets are great for those who have diabetes as they contain a number of phytonutrients that provide strong anti-inflammatory benefits. In addition to this, a certain pigment in the beet known as betalin is also known to help to provide strong detoxification benefits, so that's yet another clear advantage to include them in your diet. By detoxifying your system you'll feel and function better on a day to day basis. Finally, even though beets are considered high glycemic they are also very rich in fiber so will provide blood sugar control after eating them with your meal.

BELL PEPPERS

Our next vegetable that's well known for the antioxidant benefits it provides is bell peppers. The antioxidants in this food can help with those suffering from diabetes and can also help to prevent cardiovascular disease development. For those who are battling excess weight with their diabetes, bell peppers contain a certain phytonutrient known as capsaicin, which can increase the metabolic rate after consumption. This means that you'll burn more calories throughout the day, thus improving your chances at weight loss. Bell peppers are also very rich sources of vitamin C and A, providing over 100% of your total daily requirements.

BLACK BEANS

Beans are often linked to a lower overall development of Type 2 diabetes, and for those who are currently suffering, they're a great food for helping to gain better control over the condition. Black beans are very high in both protein and fiber, which offers a double protection against spiking blood glucose levels. There are also special enzymes in black beans, alpha-amylase enzymes which help to slow the breakdown of starch into sugar in the body, further enhancing the blood-glucose control they provide you. Start adding these to your diet today.

BLACKBERRIES

Blackberries are a fruit that has a very high antioxidant concentration so will help to provide anti-oxidant and anti-inflammatory protection. In addition to this, this berry is one of the highest fiber containing berries, so will really slow down the blood glucose response you get after eating it.

BLUEBERRIES

If there's one fruit you must include in your diet, blueberries are it. Blueberries rank very low on the GI index scale, so will provide much help with blood sugar regulation for those suffering from Type 2 diabetes. Blueberries have also been known to help boost your memory ability, so are especially helpful in those who are aging and experiencing memory declines. Blueberries are rich in vitamin C and manganese as well and provide just 81 calories per cup. As a study published by the United States Department of Agriculture noted, blueberries are one of the top sources of antioxidants that can help to reduce the development of metabolic syndrome and diabetes. Toss them into your yogurt, a bowl of oatmeal, or eat them on their own as a quick snack.

BROCCOLI

One of the most commonly consumed vegetables that you'll want to be sure you're taking in is broccoli. Broccoli is very low in calories at just 43 per cup so is easy to add into the diet of a diabetic who is watching their weight. Broccoli is also rich in a number of nutrients including vitamin C, K, A, folate, potassium, vitamin B6 and B2, phosphorus, and magnesium.

Broccoli will also supply a small dose of iron and calcium, two minerals that are imperative to strong bones and high energy levels. Those who consume broccoli as part of their regular diet enjoy reduction in chronic inflammation and protection against oxidative stress.

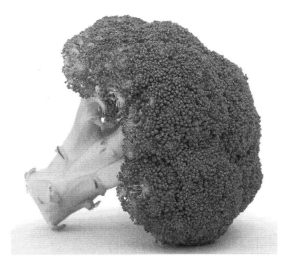

BROWN RICE

Brown rice is very well known for its manganese content, as just a one cup serving will provide you with 88% of your total daily value. This mineral is heavily involved in helping the body derive energy from proteins and carbohydrates that are consumed, so will help ensure that you maintain high energy levels. In addition to this, whole grains such as brown rice are believed to help reduce the risk of insulin resistance, which is heavily associated with diabetes.

BRUSSELS SPROUTS

Another commonly overlooked vegetable that you should start reconsidering is Brussels sprouts. This vegetable is also remarkable for the anti-inflammatory effects it has on the body, so is great for those with any inflammatory condition such as Type 2 diabetes, inflammatory bowel disease, or rheumatoid arthritis. Brussels sprouts are also excellent for promoting better digestion as they contain over 4 grams of fiber per cup, so will ensure the smooth passage of food through your track. Finally, this vegetable is also very effective for helping to lower the levels of cholesterol in the body, so if you're suffering from high cholesterol levels one to strongly consider.

BUCKWHEAT

One whole grain that many people never even think about having is buckwheat. It's time to put this food back into your diet however as it's one of the healthiest, energy-producing carbohydrate sources around. The nutrient combination in buckwheat, especially the chiro-inositol compound found in it, will help to control blood sugar levels more than those from refined wheat flours, so will be perfect for stabilizing your glucose level and increasing your satiety from the meal.

CABBAGE

The next food that's a must-have on the diabetic's meal plan is cabbage. Cabbage is one of the most nutrient dense vegetables around and at a mere 33 calories per cup serving, it's also an easy add to your diet plan. Cabbage supplies close to 100% of your total vitamin K requirement, and is also a great source of vitamin C, manganese, vitamin B6, folate, and potassium. Cabbage is especially well known for helping to prevent the development of cancer, but it will also help provide anti-inflammatory support to anyone suffering from a related inflammatory condition such as Type 2 diabetes. Be sure to include both green and red varieties in your diet for best results.

CANTALOUPE

One melon that's excellent for the health benefits it provides is cantaloupe. This fruit is extremely high in vitamin C content, which is going to help keep your immune system in proper working order to help reduce the chance of the common cold or other viruses. Cantaloupe is also very high in a number of B-vitamins, which play a key role in the release of carbohydrates in the body while maintaining steady blood sugar levels. For the diabetic, this is a particularly good advantage.

CARROTS

Another cancer fighting vegetable to add to your diet is carrots. Carrots are very high in beta-carotene and will help to reduce the risk of cardiovascular disease and will also help to support proper vision due to their high carotenoid content. Carrots also pack in a good dose of fiber in every serving, so will also help to keep your blood sugar levels regulated when added to your meal. Toss them into a salad for extra blood sugar regulating effects.

CASHEWS

One other nut that should make its way into your diet is the cashew. Cashews do contain less fat than some other nut varieties, but of the fat they contain, 75% of it is the unsaturated variety. In addition to this, they're also high in oleic acid, which is a type of fat that can help promote better heart health in those with diabetes. By adding these to your diet you can decrease the amount of triglycerides present, which is a key risk factor for the development of heart disease. Cashews are a very rich source of magnesium, which will help to promote strong bones and proper muscular contractions in the body as well. Keep in mind that a serving of any nut is approximately ¼ cup.

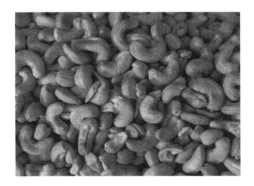

CAULIFLOWER

One great vegetable to add as a side dish to your meals is cauliflower. This vegetable is rich in glucosinolates and isothiocyanates that will provide strong anti-inflammatory protection to those suffering from diabetes. Cauliflower is also high in vitamin K and omega-3 fatty acids, which provide further inflammatory support and can reduce your risk of cardiovascular disease. This vegetable is low in calories at just 28 per cup, so make sure you add it into your diet today.

CAYENNE PEPPER

Since weight control is very important to those with diabetes, looking at adding cayenne pepper into your recipes is a wise move. This spice can help to increase the metabolism after consumption so that you burn calories at an accelerated rate, assisting weight loss and weight control. In addition to that, it can also help to enhance your overall immunity.

CELERY

If there's one vegetable that's low in calories, celery would be it. Coming in with just 19 calories per cup, this vegetable is excellent to add extra bulk to your meal and provide you with a number of nutrients to promote good health. Since weight control is such an important aspect of dealing with diabetes, adding celery frequently will help maintaining that low calorie diet easier. Celery is high in vitamin K and vitamin C and will help to keep your immune system strong while reducing blood pressure. Celery also acts as a natural diuretic in the body and can help to regulate your fluid balance for optimal health.

CHICKEN

One of the top protein sources that you can eat, chicken should also be added to your diet if you have diabetes. Chicken is low in saturated fat and very high in fiber, so will break down slowly in the body having very little influence over blood glucose levels. Chicken is especially high in selenium, which is a trace mineral that will help to provide antioxidant protection and help to boost your immune system as well.

CHILI PEPPER

Just like cayenne pepper, chilli peppers are going to help to increase the metabolism after a meal and will quickly increase your total daily calorie burn. Furthermore, most individuals will consume less food total in a meal that is spicier, so the addition of this to your meal could decrease the total amount of food that you consume, thus providing even further weight reduction benefits.

CILANTRO

Another spice not to be forgotten, Cilantro can also help to control blood sugar levels and stimulate the natural release of insulin in the body. One study also found that cilantro can help to reduce triglyceride levels in addition to blood glucose levels in those with diabetes.

CINNAMON

One sweet spice that you'll definitely want to be sure to add into your diet is cinnamon. Cinnamon is excellent for helping to control blood sugar levels after carbohydrates are consumed. One study published by the American Diabetes Association noted that 1, 3, and 6 grams of cinnamon per day all reduced serum glucose levels, blood triglyceride levels, LDL Cholesterol, as well as total cholesterol levels in those with diabetes.

CLOVES

If you're already eating a diet full of foods that reduce inflammation in the body, adding cloves to your diet can enhance those benefits even further. The addition of this spice can decrease inflammation by another 15-30% over and above what you'd experience with your food choices alone.

COD

Cod fish is an excellent source of low-fat protein that will really help the diabetic maintain maximum blood glucose control and meet their protein requirements for the day. Cod is also rich in vitamin B6, vitamin B12, and omega-3 fatty acids, all of which will provide strong cardiovascular benefits. Eating this fish just a few times a week can help to lower your triglyceride levels and keep heart disease in check.

COLLARD GREENS

Collard Greens are a form of cruciferous vegetable that many people don't think about when shopping at the grocery store but that add many health benefits to your diet. Like many other vegetables, these are also rich in glucosinolates and isothiocyanates, which will help to reduce the inflammation that's associated with diabetes. In addition to this, this vegetable is a fiber powerhouse, packing in five grams with each cup that you eat. This is perfect for those who are seeking digestive support. Finally, this food can help to provide detoxification benefits, flushing toxins from your system that would otherwise cause harm.

CORN

Corn is a vegetable that is higher in calories than others and considered high glycemic. However at 4.6 grams of fiber per cup, corn is a good fiber source and shouldn't be excluded from your diet. According to the non-profit George Mateljan Foundation, consumption of corn in ordinary amounts has been shown to be associated with better blood sugar control in both Type 1 and Type 2 diabetes. A great source of antioxidants and rich in thiamine, corn is a great food to add as a side dish to your protein source.

COTTAGE CHEESE

Cottage cheese is a high protein, lower fat dairy product that you should include in your diet. Those that include more dairy products in their daily diet tend to see greater weight loss in the abdominal region, which is key for keeping your body healthy and warding off insulin resistance.

CRANBERRIES

Providing both anti-inflammatory and anti-cancer benefits, cranberries are a juicy fruit that you should dig into. Cranberries are also well-known for their ability to help ward off urinary tract infection, so if that's a concern for you, something that you'll definitely want to note. In addition to this, cranberries provide strong immune support due to the proanthocyanidins that they contain. Whether you choose to drink the juice or eat the fruit itself, you'll reap all these benefits and more. Researchers from the University of Maine also noted that 200 ml of juice per day taken for 3 months lowered the overall fasting blood glucose level in those who had Type 2 diabetes.

CUCUMBERS

While cucumbers are made mostly of water, they are an excellent addition to your diet plan. At just 13 calories per cup, you can literally fill up on as many of these as you'd like without risking weight gain or an increase to your blood sugar level. When you're craving a crunchy snack, choose cucumbers over higher carb items such as potato chips or crackers.

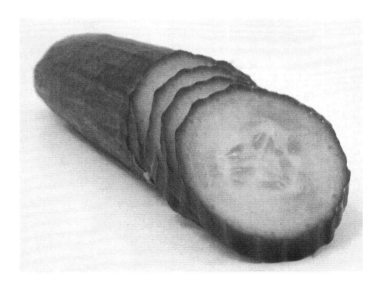

EGGPLANT

Eggplant is a vegetable that ranks low on the GI scale so will be a good food for those who are trying to control their blood sugar level. This food is rich in phenolic antioxidant compounds, which will help to reduce oxidative stress on the body that lead to disease. In addition to that, this food is great for providing a high level of cardiovascular health support, so can protect against any problems associated with your cardiovascular system.

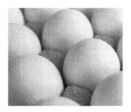

EGGS

A can't-beat breakfast protein source (or any meal for that matter), eggs are high in tryptophan, selenium, iodine, and riboflavin. They're also rich in choline, which will help lower the level of chronic inflammation in the body, which proves to be especially helpful for those with diabetes. Eggs have long been considered the most complete source of protein because they contain sufficient amounts of all the essential amino acids the body requires. They can be prepared numerous ways: fried, scrambled, poached, boiled, deviled, in an omelet, used in a salad, or in a quiche. Be creative!

FENNEL

Fennel is another overlooked vegetable to start adding to your diet. This vegetable works great sautéed or added into a salad and offers powerful antioxidant protection and immune system support thanks to its high vitamin C content. Another fiber-powerhouse, this vegetable will also help to control blood sugar levels as it increases the time of digestion.

FIGS

and more notably, Fig Leaves

While figs only come around at certain points in the year, you can get dried figs year round and they are an excellent addition to your diet plan. Figs are very high in dietary fiber content and also contain a good dose of potassium as well as manganese. What's especially notable about figs is that the fig leaf may help to lower the amount of insulin required by those with diabetes. Simply adding fig leaf extract to some of your dishes will provide this effect, so start considering this on some occasions.

FLAXSEED OIL

Just like flaxseeds, flaxseed oil is also an excellent addition to your diet and works great in replacement of other oils in a variety of dishes. Flaxseed oil will be a very concentrated form of omega-fats, more so than the seeds which also contain the added fiber and carbs, so is great for those who really want to watch their carbohydrate intake.

FLAXSEEDS

For optimal health and disease protection, you must consider adding flaxseeds to your diet. Flaxseeds are rich in omega-3 fats, which will help to reduce insulin resistance. In addition to that, the omega-fats will also provide clear anti-inflammatory benefits and will also contain a moderate dose of protein and fiber as well. Sprinkle them onto yogurt or oatmeal or grind them and consider adding them to your baking.

GARLIC

One spice that you should start using more often if you already aren't is garlic. Garlic is rich in flavonoids and suflur-containing nutrients that will help to boost your cardiovascular health, lower blood pressure, and provide anti-inflammatory benefits that assist with the prevention and treatment of any inflammatory condition including diabetes. To enhance the health benefits garlic provides, use it chopped or crushed as this makes it more potent overall.

GINGER

Ginger is spice that will quickly boost the flavor of your foods so that you don't have to add high-sugar condiments or sauces. In addition to this, it contains compounds known as gingerols that will provide anti-inflammatory benefits for the body. Those who include this in their diet also show signs of an enhanced immune system as well.

GRAPEFRUIT

One fruit that's well known for its low calorie content thanks to the popular Grapefruit Diet is also wise to include on your diabetes diet. Grapefruit ranks low on the GI index and is a very powerful vitamin C rich fruit that will help to boost your immune system while preventing heart disease and stroke.

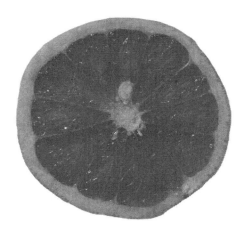

GRAPES

Also ranking in low on the GI index scale with a value of 49, grapes are a perfect sweet treat when your cravings strike. Grapes are very rich in manganese and also contain vitamin C, vitamin B1, potassium, and vitamin B6. This fruit is very high in flavonoid content that can help to protect LDL cholesterol from free radical damage and improve your heart health.

GREEK YOGURT

Greek yogurt is one of the healthiest yogurts that you could add to your diet as a diabetic as it's very low in sugar, fat free, and contains a very high amount of protein. Pair this with some fresh berries and flaxseeds or sliced almonds for the perfect snack to help control your blood sugar levels.

GREEN BEANS

As far as helping those with diabetes, green beans have two important things going for them: a very high fiber level and strong carotenoid and flavonoid content. Together these two factors help to reduce the inflammation in the body and help those with diabetes manage their condition better. Green beans are also a lower calorie option to add to your diet so are perfect for those seeking weight control.

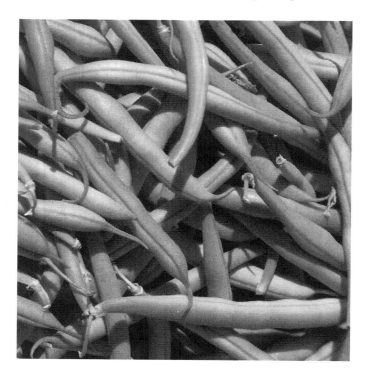

GREEN PEAS

Like corn, green peas do contain more overall calories and carbohydrates than some other vegetables do, but they are also an excellent way to reduce inflammation in the body and improve your control over diabetes. Green peas are a very good source of vitamin K, manganese, vitamin C, vitamin B1, folate, vitamin A, phosphorus, vitamin B3 and B6, as well as iron and zinc. With such a stellar nutrient line-up, you'd be missing out if you didn't include these in your diet plan. You will experience the best flavor in frozen or fresh green peas.

GREEN TEA

Green tea is the next addition to your diet to consider. Hot fluids will have a natural appetite soothing effect on the body and green tea in particular can help to improve insulin sensitivity in those who are suffering from Type 2 diabetes.

HALIBUT

Halibut is one of the fish varieties that is very rich in omega-3 fatty acids, which can help to improve insulin sensitivity in those who are suffering from diabetes. This fish is also high in protein, selenium, as well as tryptophan, and will promote overall better cardiovascular health.

HONEYDEW

Honeydew is a sweet melon that many people enjoy that will be a great addition to your diet. This melon contains 64 calories per one cup serving and is a great source of vitamin B6, folate, potassium, and vitamin C. Together these will help maximize energy levels and help provide strong anti-oxidant support.

KALE

Kale shines for its anti-inflammatory benefits due to the high level of vitamin K found in this vegetable. It's one of the richest sources of this nutrient around, so to meet your daily intake, have a one cup serving with your salad or added into a stir-fry. The benefits of kale are intensified when you steam this vegetable, so consider this cooking method when preparing it.

KIDNEY BEANS

Kidney beans are a powerhouse food for the diabetic due to their high fiber and high protein content. These beans also contain a healthy dose of carbs, so make for a complete food to add into your diet. Those who have very high fiber diets will maintain much better blood sugar control throughout the day and experience a lower overall insulin release. The manganese found in kidney beans will also help with energy production and for providing antioxidant support.

KIWIFRUIT

If you're looking to boost your immune system and combat your cravings for something sweet yet tart at the same time, consider kiwifruit. Kiwifruit contains more vitamin C than your average orange and also offers a good dose of fiber and potassium as well. The antioxidants found in kiwifruit are going to be especially beneficial for helping to combat osteoarthritis, rheumatoid arthritis, as well for preventing conditions such as cancer and diabetic heart disease.

LEEKS

Leeks are a food that contains a very high polyphenol content, which is especially notable for those who are suffering from diabetes as it can help to improve health problems related to oxidative stress, which includes diabetes along with atherosclerosis and rheumatoid arthritis. Leeks also offer top notch cardiovascular support due to high folate levels. Start adding leeks to your dinner meal more often.

MACKEREL

Mackerel is a fish that's higher in calories than other white fish varieties but is filled with good nutrition. This fish contains more essential fatty acids than white fish does and is also high in phosphorus, vitamin D, niacin, selenium, and vitamin B12. A study from the American Journal of Clinical Nutrition noted that adding vitamin D rich foods to your diet can help with Type 1 diabetes amongst other conditions. Adding this fish to your meals can also help to slow the blood glucose response as the protein and fats slow the digestion process down.

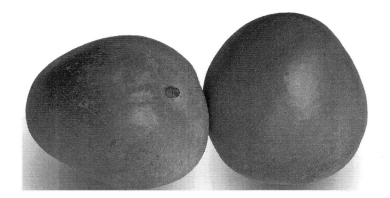

MANGO

If you're someone who enjoys exotic fruits, mango is definitely a fruit that you'll want to try out. This fruit is rich in vitamin B6, and also provides a good dose of vitamin A and C as well. Ranking in as low on the GI index scale, you can feel good about satisfying your sweet tooth with this snack that won't cause a large impact on your blood sugar levels.

MILLET

Millet is another whole grain that you should include in your diet to control diabetes. This grain contains magnesium in high levels, which will help with glucose utilization by the body and also promote proper insulin secretion. In addition to this, the magnesium will also help to promote a healthier heart by reducing heart attack and lowering blood pressure.

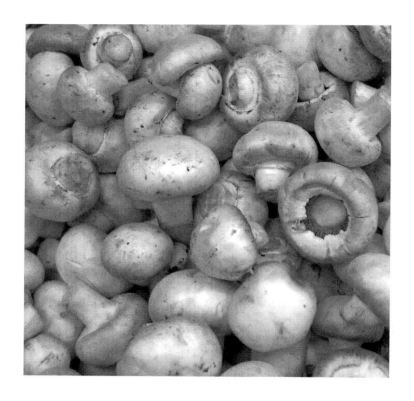

MUSHROOMS

Mushrooms are a tasty vegetable that works great in stir-fry's, salads, or just sautéed in a small amount of olive oil and garlic and will provide a number of important health benefits. Mushrooms are very powerful for providing high levels of immune system support as they help with the formation and maintenance of white blood cells. Mushrooms will also provide strong cardiovascular benefits because of their high content of B vitamins including Vitamin B2, B3, B5, B6, and B12.

MUSTARD GREENS

Mustard greens are the next cruciferous vegetable that you should think about including in your diet program. This vegetable is very high in vitamin K, vitamin A, and Vitamin C content, while also being rich in folate, manganese, and vitamin E. Mustard greens will offer detoxification benefits to the body as well as providing a strong anti-inflammatory effect so are great for those looking to improve their health with diabetes. To reap the greatest health benefits of this vegetable, allow them to sit in cool water for five minutes.

OATS

Moving on to another standout whole grain to include in your diet is oats. Oats are very rich in fiber content and contain no sugar, so will digest very slowly in the body which is precisely what a diabetic needs. Oats are also high in volume so will fill you up quickly, making it easier to maintain a lower calorie intake. Steer clear of the instant oatmeal and reach for Steel Cut or Old Fashioned Oats to reap all the benefits of this grain.

OLIVE OIL

Just as olives made the list of top healthy foods that you should be consuming, so does olive oil. Olive oil is very well known for its high level of heart health benefits and it can also help to prevent the development of cancer. Olive oil will also offer anti-inflammatory benefits as well, making it a great food for diabetics.

OLIVES

Olives are a high fat food that will help to protect your heart health and keep your blood sugar levels controlled. This food is also a very good source of iron and vitamin E, two essential nutrients for high energy levels and for reducing the amount of free radical damage in the body. Toss these onto your salad or eat them raw – whatever you prefer.

ONIONS

Onions are a vegetable that works great with stir-fry's or salads and offer numerous health benefits to the diabetic. This food comes in at just 60 calories per cup and is very high in chromium, a specific mineral that is key in stabilizing blood sugar levels. Those who suffer from chromium deficiency have impairment in their ability to use glucose to meet energy needs, therefore this can raise your insulin requirement even higher. This mineral is often used as a treatment for diabetes, so by including onions in your diet, you can take the natural approach.

ORANGES

One great low calorie food that ranks low on the GI index that you should eat to support good health is the orange. Oranges are high in fiber and vitamin C content, two essential factors that make it a perfect diabetic food choice. Their high vitamin C content will also be very beneficial for helping to promote a strong immune system and keep you illness free.

PAPAYA

Papaya's rank right up there with oranges for their high vitamin C content and for offering top notch anti-inflammatory support to those with diabetes. This fruit can also help to protect against macular degeneration (vision loss) as well as help to keep your lungs healthy.

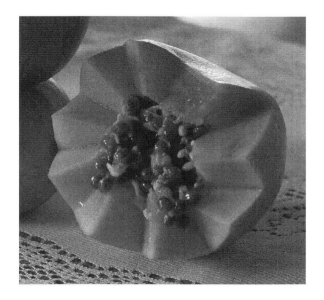

PARSLEY

Eating foods that are more Alkaline will help the diabetic control inflammation. Parsley is a free radical scavenger and has histamine inhibitors. It is rich in vitamins A, C, minerals, and other compounds that clear the toxins from the body. It not only tastes good and is used as a garnish on other foods, it also acts as a great breath freshener due to its high chlorophyll content.

PEACHES

Peaches are another of the sweeter fruits that's very high in vitamin C so will provide great anti-oxidant benefits to the body and help reduce inflammation. Peaches are also higher in fiber at 3 grams per large peach and are a good source of vitamin A, Niacin, and potassium.

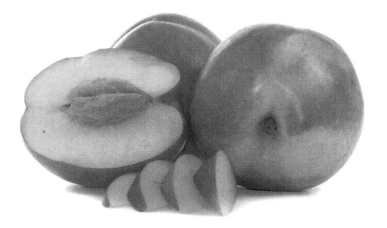

PEANUTS

One of the most commonly eaten foods that's often thought to be a nut, the peanut is actually a legume. This food is very rich in healthy fats along with manganese, tryptophan, vitamin B3, folate, copper, and even contains a small amount of protein. This makes it great for slowing down digestion and stopping hunger, so consider adding it to your meal or having it as a light snack between meals. One study published by the American Journal of Clinical Nutrition noted that the higher the incidence of legume consumption, the lower the incidence of diabetes, illustrating the strong connection with this food.

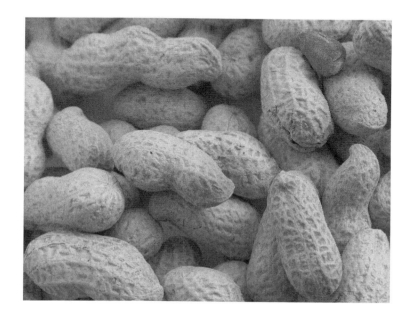

PEARS

Pears are an excellent high fiber fruit to eat to help control blood sugar levels while promoting a healthy cardiovascular system. This fruit can also offer protection against colon cancer, which is another reason to consider adding it into your diet plan.

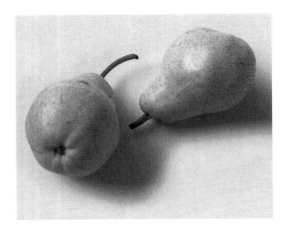

PINEAPPLE

Pineapple contains a great mixture of manganese and thiamine, which are two important nutrients that are required for proper energy development in the body. They will also help to provide top-notch antioxidant defense so can help to ward off free radical damage. This sweet treat comes in at 66 on the GI scale so moderate your portion sizes when eating it. With the added fiber it contains it's still a great food for the diabetic.

PLUMS

One standout benefit that plums have to offer is that they increase the absorption of iron in the body, therefore increasing your energy levels in an indirect way. Plums are also very high in vitamin C, so will help to protect good cholesterol from being harmed from free radicals that you may come into contact with. At 36 calories per fruit, this is a low calorie snack to have between meals.

PUMPKIN SEEDS

Another food that's high in healthy fats to consider adding to your diet plan is pumpkin seeds. Pumpkin seeds are rich in manganese, magnesium, phosphorus, tryptophan, iron, as well as copper, vitamin K, and zinc. These nutrients together can help to bring down your overall cholesterol levels and improve your immune system response. Because of their healthy fat content they'll also have a low impact on blood glucose levels.

QUINOA (keen wah)

One whole grain that is quite similar to brown rice but offers a different nutritional profile is Quinoa. Quinoa is excellent or those with diabetes as it contains a complete protein, so the impact it has on your blood glucose levels will be much lower. Quinoa is also a great source of manganese, magnesium, and iron.

RASPBERRIES

Raspberries rank in close to top spot for the antioxidant protection they deliver compared to other produce picks, providing more support than strawberries, kiwis, as well as tomatoes. In addition to the high level of ellagitannins, a specific form of antioxidant found in the raspberry, they also are rich in B vitamins, which help the body derive energy from the foods you eat. Researchers also noted in a study published by the Journal of Food Biochemistry that raspberries can help to improve hypertension management in those with diabetes.

RED PEPPERS

Red peppers as well as other bell peppers are a very potent source of anti-oxidants which can help to ward off cardiovascular disease and also aid those with diabetes. Red peppers are low in calories at only 24 per cup, so they will be an easy food to add into your diet. Rich in vitamin C and vitamin A, they'll also help to keep your immune system strong.

ROMAINE LETTUCE

If you're preparing a salad, one thing that you must do is swap out your iceberg lettuce for some romaine instead. Romaine lettuce is much higher in vitamin K content and is also a very rich source of vitamin A, vitamin C, folate, manganese, chromium, and potassium. As we discovered with onions, the chromium content along makes this a must-have food on the diabetic's checklist for regulating the blood sugar-insulin response.

RYE

If you're looking for top-notch hunger support, turn to rye. Rye is very high in noncellulose polysaccharides, which help to increase the amount of water it binds with, making it provoke very high levels of satiety in the body after eating it. Due to this high fiber content, you'll get a much lower blood glucose response from rye bread than whole wheat bread, so consider making the switch over to rye instead.

SALMON

Salmon is a top notch protein source of the diabetic due to the high level of essential fats it contains as well as the high protein and vitamin D content. Salmon is also high in selenium and vitamin B3 and B12, so will help you maintain high energy levels. The omega-fats found in salmon will enhance insulin sensitivity so you maintain better blood glucose control.

SESAME SEEDS

The major nutrients that are found in high concentrations in sesame seeds include copper, manganese, tryptophan, calcium, and magnesium. Sesame seeds are also a great source of healthy fats, so will help to control blood sugar levels after a mixed meal is eaten. Sesame seeds can also help to reduce your cholesterol levels, promoting good heart health as well.

SHRIMP

Shrimp is a very low calorie form of protein that is perfect for a quick addition to round out your meals. Shrimp does contain small amounts of omega-3 fatty acids, which help to increase your sensitivity to glucose. Additionally, those who consume their essential fatty acids from foods rather than strictly from supplements tend to note better overall health benefits, making shrimp an excellent choice.

SOYBEANS

Soybeans are an excellent addition to your diet due to the combination of fiber and protein that they provide. Since two keys to maximizing blood glucose levels are eating enough protein and fiber together, this food has it all. Soybeans also help to promote lower cholesterol levels and prevent heart disease, which is of particular concern to those who suffer from diabetes.

SPELT

One grain that you very rarely ever hear of is spelt, however if you're a diabetic this is one to consider adding to your diet program. Spelt is high in fiber and also rich in magnesium, which can help to reduce the risk or symptoms associated with Type 2 diabetes. Spelt is also high in niacin, which can help to reduce the risk of atherosclerosis development.

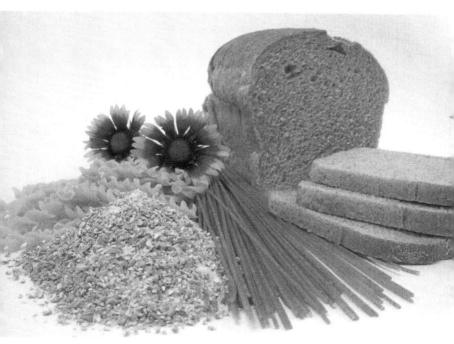

SPINACH

Spinach is a very healthy alternative to use in place of lettuce with your salads and is perfect for increasing your iron intake. Spinach is also an excellent source of phytonutrients, which will provide clear anti-inflammatory support, reducing symptoms of diabetes and helping to protect against cancer. Finally, the vitamin K content in spinach is very helpful in promoting strong bones, so ideal for those who want to maintain good bone health.

STRAWBERRIES

Strawberries are a favored berry among many and fit perfectly in the diabetic's diet. They're low in calories at just 43 per cup and contain plenty of vitamin C, manganese, as well as dietary fiber. Strawberries will have very little impact on your blood sugar levels and are a perfect way to control your craving for something sweet.

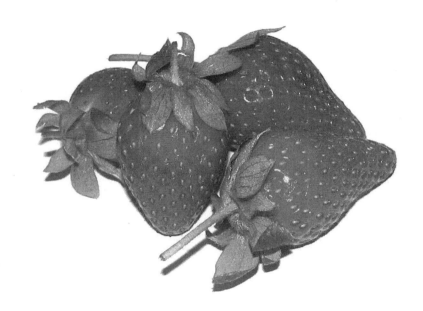

SUMMER SQUASH

Summer squash has a form of carbohydrates called polysaccharides that are especially rich in D-galacturonic acid that help to provide enhanced insulin regulation. Kathleen Melanson from the Department of Nutrition and Food Sciences noted that summer squash amongst other unrefined plant foods can help to combat insulin resistance. This food is also a relatively low calorie food coming in at only 36 calories per one cup serving, so it's an excellent addition to any diabetic's diet who is looking to maximize weight loss or maintain their weight.

SUNFLOWER SEEDS

To add flavor to your next salad, consider topping it with sunflower seeds. These seeds are high in healthy fats and will help to slow the digestion process, keeping your blood sugar levels stable. They're also a very good source of vitamin E, which will provide strong cardiovascular disease protection.

SWEET POTATOES

Many people with diabetes think they must fear all potatoes, but this isn't the case when it comes to sweet potatoes. If boiled or steamed they will have a GI index value of just 50, making them rate low on the scale. In addition to this, sweet potatoes can help to increase the blood levels of adiponectin in the body, which is a hormone that helps to moderate insulin metabolism providing diabetics with even better blood glucose control.

SWISS CHARD

Swiss chard is a particular vegetable that the diabetic should pay close attention to. This vegetable contains a unique flavonoid that can help to prevent the rapid break-down of carbohydrates into sugar in the blood, therefore it will really help to keep blood sugar levels stable. In addition to this, this vegetable is an excellent source of vitamin C, E, and beta-carotene.

TEMPEH

Tempeh, like soybeans contains both protein and fiber in one food, which you'd never find in many other meat-based protein sources. This provides high levels of control over your blood sugar level while also adding the benefit of lowering LDL levels in the body. For anyone who is a vegetarian, this food is a must. Researchers from the Beltsville Human Nutrition Research Center noted that soy protein can help to reduce serum insulin and insulin resistance in those who suffer from diabetes.

TOFU

If you aren't a fan of tempeh and are looking for a non-meat protein to include in your diet, consider tofu. The soy protein in tofu can help to lower LDL levels while increasing HDL levels, therefore reducing the level of harmful triglycerides in the blood stream. These can really cause problems for diabetic patients who are at risk for heart disease, so an important benefit to take note of.

TOMATOES

Tomatoes and tomato juice is of particular importance for diabetics as it can help to improve blood clotting abilities. This is an issue that some diabetics do need to be concerned with as their blood vessels can be impaired which reduces the ability of the blood to clot. Adding tomatoes to the diet can prevent this.

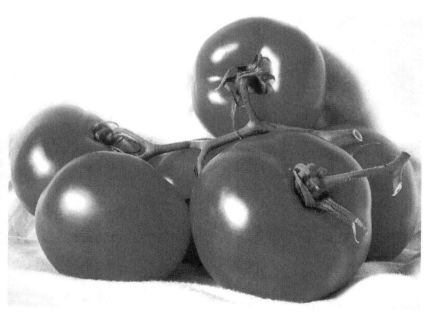

TUNA

One very lean source of protein to consider adding to your diet is tuna. Tuna is rich in selenium, tryptophan, as well as niacin, vitamin B6, and vitamin B1 and will easily help you meet your daily protein requirements. Tuna is also rich in omega-3 fats, which can help to prevent obesity and help improve the insulin response in the body.

TURKEY

Turkey is another great way to meet your protein requirements and help stabilize blood sugars with a meal containing carbohydrates. Those who consume a high amount of red meat in their diet are more likely to suffer from conditions such as heart disease and Type 2 diabetes, so turkey offers relief from red meat as it's a white variation.

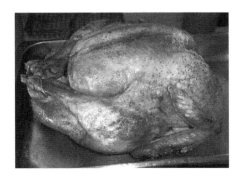

TURMERIC

One spice that you should definitely consider adding to your diet plan is turmeric. This spice contains a molecule known as curcumin, which can help to lower the levels of LDL in the body, reducing your risk of cardiovascular disease. This spice can also help to enhance the health of the liver and prevent colon cancer development.

TURNIP GREENS

Turnip greens are an excellent source of fiber with over 5 grams per cup yet are extremely low in calories coming in at a measly 28 per serving. They're also high in vitamin K, A, and C, so will provide anti-inflammatory and anti-oxidant protection. Finally, they have sulfur-containing nutrients that will help to provide clear detoxification benefits.

VENISON

Venison is a protein source that's very rich in B vitamins and is also high in iron and phosphorus content. Since it is very low in saturated fat, this is helpful for the diabetic trying to keep their total cholesterol levels under control and maintain a healthy weight.

WALNUTS

Walnuts are very rich in omega-fats and perfect for calming your appetite. It's also high in manganese and tryptophan, while being great for those with Type 2 diabetes as they will help to lower the risk of cardiovascular problems. Researchers from the University of Wollongong found that diabetics who increased their intake to 30 grams of walnuts per day achieved significantly greater increases in HDL cholesterol to total cholesterol in their body.

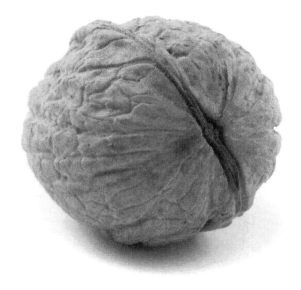

WATERMELON

Watermelon is another great food that has anti-inflammatory benefits and can help to battle against conditions such as high blood pressure, atherosclerosis and colon cancer. Watermelon is full of anti-oxidants and B-vitamins which will support high energy levels in the body. But be cautious with Watermelon because it is high glycemic. Three-quarters of a cup of watermelon balls has fewer than nine grams of carbohydrates which can be a safe serving for many diabetics.

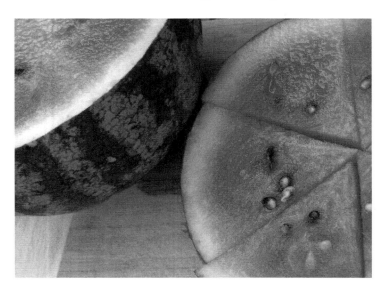

WINTER SQUASH

The antioxidant and anti-inflammatory compounds in winter squash make this tasty starch-like vegetable a «super-star» among "starchy" vegetables. Supplying more than a days worth of Vitamin A, it is rich in carotenoids and is a surprising source of important Omega 3 fatty acids. An increasing number of animal studies now show that winter squash also have anti-diabetic and insulin-regulating properties. Some common varieties of winter squash include Butternut Squash, Acorn Squash, Hubbard Squash, Turan Squash and Kabocha Squash.

So there you have it – 101 foods that can help you manage your diabetes. Including the most varied selection of foods in your daily diet is the single best way to stay on track and make sure that you're getting all the wholesome nutrition you need. So be sure to change up your meal plan regularly.

Any of the above foods will offer numerous benefits to help control your blood sugar level, strengthen your immune system, and keep you feeling your best. Now go to the **Handy List for Shopping for The 101 Best Diabetic Foods** to start making your list for your next grocery trip.

GET THE LATEST DIABETES RESEARCH AND CLINICALLY PROVEN METHODS THAT THE BIG PHARMACEUTICAL COMPANIES DON'T WANT YOU TO KNOW TO CURE YOUR DIABETES NATURALLY.

DiabeticDoctor.com

Handy List for Shopping for The 101 Best Diabetic Foods

Below you will find the foods listed in a section where you might find them in a grocery store. Some items may be found in more than one place in your store so that is why you will find them listed in more than one section below. Whenever possible ... eat FRESH ... not canned or preserved. Enjoy!

FRESH FRUITS and VEGETABLES

Apples
Apricots
Asparagus
Avocados
Bananas
Basil
Beets
Bell Peppers
Blackberries
Blueberries
Broccoli
Brussels Sprouts
Cabbage
Cantaloupe
Carrots
Cauliflower
Celery
Chili Pepper
Cilantro
Collard Greens
Corn
Cranberries
Cucumbers
Eggplant
Figs And More
Notably,
Fig Leaves
Fennel
Garlic
Ginger
Grapefruit
Grapes
Green Beans
Green Peas
Honeydew

Kale
Kiwifruit
Leeks
Mango
Mushrooms
Mustard Greens
Onions
Oranges
Papaya
Parsley
Peaches
Pears
Pineapple
Plums
Raspberries
Red Peppers
Romaine Lettuce
Spinach
Strawberries
Summer Squash
Sweet Potatoes
Swiss Chard
Tomatoes
Turnip Greens
Watermelon
Winter Squash

REFRIGERATED / DAIRY CASE
Cottage Cheese
Eggs
Greek Yogurt
Tofu

FRESH MEAT CASE
Beef, Lean
Chicken
Cod
Halibut
Mackerel
Salmon
Shrimp
Tuna
Turkey
Venison

FROZEN CASE
Cranberries
Green Tea
Green Beans
Green Peas

CEREAL AISLE
Barley
Brown Rice
Buckwheat
Millet
Oats

SPICE AISLE
Cayenne Pepper
Chili Pepper
Cinnamon
Cloves
Garlic
Ginger
Turmeric
Flaxseed Oil
Olive Oil

NUTS
Almonds
Cashews
Flaxseeds
Peanuts
Pumpkin Seeds
Sesame Seeds
Soybeans
Sunflower Seeds
Walnuts

DRIED LENTILS/ CANNED VEGETABLES
Black Beans
Kidney Beans
Tomatoes

CONDIMENT AISLE
Olives

TEA AISLE
Green Tea

HEALTH FOOD SECTION or HEALTH FOOD STORE
Buckwheat
Millet
Oats
Quinoa
Rye
Spelt
Tempeh
Flaxseeds
Soybeans
Flaxseed Oil

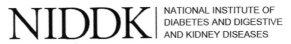

Important Diabetes Information From

NIDDK | NATIONAL INSTITUTE OF DIABETES AND DIGESTIVE AND KIDNEY DISEASES

National Diabetes Information Clearinghouse

Prevent Diabetes Problems:
Keep Your Heart and Blood Vessels Healthy

What are diabetes problems?

Too much glucose in the blood for a long time can cause diabetes problems. This high blood glucose, also called blood sugar, can damage many parts of the body, such as the heart, blood vessels, eyes, and kidneys. Heart and blood vessel disease can lead to heart attacks and strokes, the leading causes of death for people with diabetes. You can do a lot to prevent or slow down diabetes problems.

This booklet is about heart and blood vessel problems caused by diabetes. You will learn the things you can do each day and during each year to stay healthy and prevent diabetes problems.

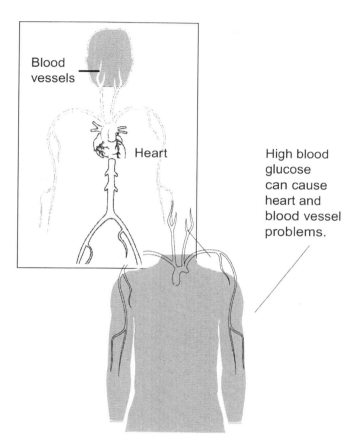

Blood vessels

Heart

High blood glucose can cause heart and blood vessel problems.

What should I do each day to stay healthy with diabetes?

Follow the healthy eating plan that you and your doctor or dietitian have worked out.

 Be active a total of 30 minutes most days. Ask your doctor what activities are best for you.

 Take your medicines as directed.

 Check your blood glucose every day. Each time you check your blood glucose, write the number in your record book.

 Check your feet every day for cuts, blisters, sores, swelling, redness, or sore toenails.

 Brush and floss your teeth every day.

 Control your blood pressure and cholesterol.

 Don't smoke.

What do my heart and blood vessels do?

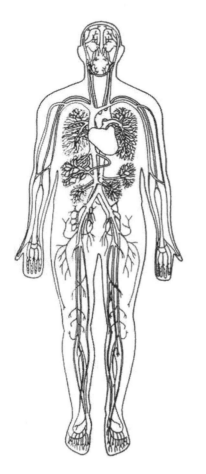

Your heart and blood vessels make up your **circulatory** system. Your heart is a muscle that pumps blood through your body. Your heart pumps blood carrying oxygen to large blood vessels, called **arteries**, and small blood vessels, called **capillaries**. Other blood vessels, called veins, carry blood back to the heart.

What can I do to prevent heart disease and stroke?

You can do a lot to prevent heart disease and stroke.

- Keep your blood glucose under control. You can see if your blood glucose is under control by having an A1C test at least twice a year. The A1C test tells you your average blood glucose for the past 2 to 3 months. The target for most people with diabetes is below 7. In some people with heart disease or other special circumstances, their doctor may recommend slightly higher levels of A1C.

- Keep your blood pressure under control. Have it checked at every doctor visit. The target for most people with diabetes is below 130/80.

- Keep your cholesterol under control. Have it checked at least once a year. The targets for most people with diabetes are

  o LDL—bad—cholesterol: below 100

  o HDL—good—cholesterol: above 40 in men and above 50 in women

  o Triglycerides — another type of fat in the blood: below 150

- Make physical activity a part of your daily routine. Aim for at least 30 minutes of exercise most days of the week. Check with your doctor to learn what activities are best for you. Take a half-hour walk every day. Or walk for 10 minutes after each meal. Use the stairs instead of the elevator. Park at the far end of the lot.

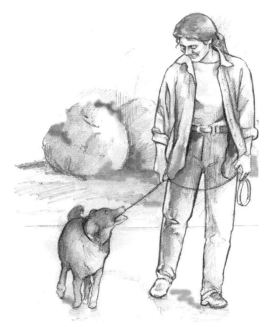

Choose an activity you like and stay active.

- Make sure the foods you eat are "heart-healthy." Include foods high in fiber, such as oat bran, oatmeal, whole-grain breads and cereals, fruits, and vegetables. Cut back on foods high in saturated fat or cholesterol, such as meats, butter, dairy products with fat, eggs, shortening, lard, and foods with palm oil or coconut oil. Limit foods with trans fat, such as snack foods and commercial baked goods.

- Lose weight if you need to. If you are overweight, try to exercise most days of the week. See a registered dietitian for help in planning meals and lowering the fat and calorie content of your diet to reach and maintain a healthy weight.

- If you smoke, quit. Your doctor can tell you about ways to help you quit smoking.

- Ask your doctor whether you should take an aspirin every day. Studies have shown that taking a low dose of aspirin every day can help reduce your risk of heart disease and stroke.

- Take your medicines as directed.

How do my blood vessels get clogged?

Several things, including having diabetes, can make your blood cholesterol level too high. Cholesterol is a substance that is made by the body and used for many important functions. Cholesterol is also found in some food derived from animals. When cholesterol is too high, the insides of large blood vessels become narrowed or clogged. This problem is called **atherosclerosis**.

Narrowed and clogged blood vessels make it harder for enough blood to get to all parts of your body. This condition can cause problems.

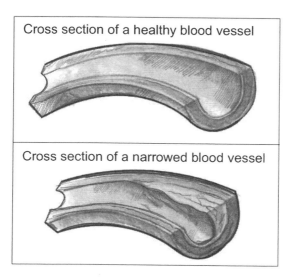

Cross section of a healthy blood vessel

Cross section of a narrowed blood vessel

What can happen when blood vessels are clogged?

When blood vessels become narrowed and clogged, you can have serious health problems:

- Chest pain, also called angina. When you have angina, you feel pain in your chest, arms, shoulders, or back. You may feel the pain more when your heart beats faster, such as when you exercise. The pain may go away when you rest. You also may sweat a lot and feel very weak. If you do not get treatment, chest pain may happen more often. If diabetes has damaged your heart nerves, you may not feel the chest pain. If you have chest pain with activity, contact your doctor.

- Heart attack. A heart attack happens when a blood vessel in or near your heart becomes blocked. Then your heart muscle can't get enough blood. When an area of your heart muscle stops working, your heart becomes weaker. During a heart attack, you may have chest pain along with nausea, indigestion, extreme weakness, and sweating. Or you may have no symptoms at all. If you have chest pain that persists, call 911. Delay in getting treatment may make a heart attack worse.

- Stroke. A stroke can happen when the blood supply to your brain is blocked. Then your brain can be damaged.

What are the warning signs of a heart attack?

You may have one or more of the following warning signs:

- chest pain or discomfort
- pain or discomfort in your arms, back, jaw, or neck
- indigestion or stomach pain
- shortness of breath
- sweating
- nausea
- light-headedness

Or, you may have no warning signs at all. Warning signs may come and go. If you have any of these warning signs, call 911 right away. Getting prompt treatment can reduce damage to the heart.

How do narrowed blood vessels cause high blood pressure?

Narrowed blood vessels leave a smaller opening for blood to flow through. Having narrowed blood vessels is like turning on a garden hose and holding your thumb over the opening. The smaller opening makes the water shoot out with more pressure.

In the same way, narrowed blood vessels lead to high blood pressure. Other factors, such as kidney problems and being overweight, also can lead to high blood pressure.

Many people with diabetes also have high blood pressure. If you have heart, eye, or kidney problems from diabetes, high blood pressure can make them worse.

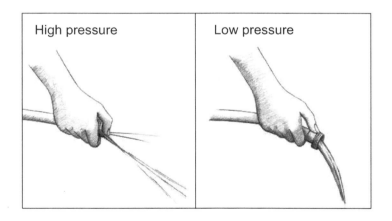

82

A smaller opening in a garden hose makes the water pressure higher. In the same way, clogged blood vessels lead to high blood pressure.

You will see your blood pressure written with two numbers separated by a slash. For example, your reading might be 120/70, said as "120 over 70." For people with diabetes, the target is to keep the first number below 130 and the second number below 80.

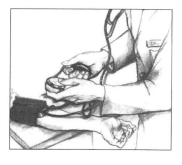

If you have high blood pressure, ask your doctor how to lower it. Your doctor may ask you to take blood pressure medicine every day. Some types of blood pressure medicine can also help keep your kidneys healthy.

You may also be able to control your blood pressure by

- eating more fruits and vegetables
- eating less salt and high-sodium foods
- losing weight if you need to
- being physically active
- not smoking
- limiting alcoholic drinks

to lower blood pressure, get to a healthy weight.

What are the warning signs of a stroke?

A stroke happens when part of your brain is not getting enough blood and stops working. Depending on the part of the brain that is damaged, a stroke can cause

- sudden weakness or numbness of your face, arm, or leg on one side of your body

- sudden confusion, trouble talking, or trouble understanding

- sudden dizziness, loss of balance, or trouble walking

- sudden trouble seeing in one or both eyes or sudden double vision

- sudden severe headache

Sometimes, one or more of these warning signs may happen and then disappear. You might be having a "mini-stroke," also called a TIA or a transient ischemic attack. If you have any of these warning signs, call 911 right away. Getting care for a TIA may reduce or prevent a stroke. Getting prompt treatment for a stroke can reduce the damage to the brain and improve chances for recovery.

How can clogged blood vessels hurt my legs and feet?

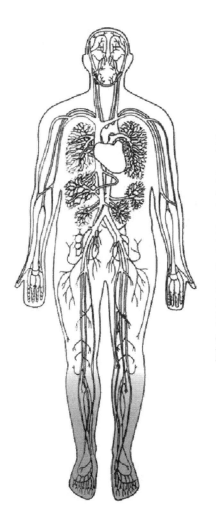

Peripheral arterial disease, also called PAD, can happen when the openings in your blood vessels become narrow and your legs and feet don't get enough blood. You may feel pain in your legs when you walk or exercise. Some people also have numbness or tingling in their feet or legs or have sores that heal slowly.

What can I do to prevent or control PAD?

- Don't smoke.

- Keep your blood glucose and blood pressure under control.

- Keep your blood fat levels close to normal.

- Be physically active.

- Ask your doctor if you should take aspirin every day.

You also may need surgery to treat PAD.

Pronunciation Guide

angina (an-JY-nuh)

arteries (AR-tur-eez)

atherosclerosis (ATH-ur-oh-sklur-OH-siss)

capillaries (KAP-ih-lair-eez)

circulatory (SUR-kyoo-luh-TOR-ee)

peripheral arterial disease
(puh-RIF-ur-uhl) (ar-TEE-ree-uhl)
(dih-ZEEZ)

transient ischemic attack
(TRANZ-see-uhnt) (iss-KEE-mik)
(uh-TAK)

For More Information

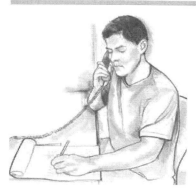

Diabetes Teachers
(nurses, dietitians, pharmacists, and other health professionals)

To find a diabetes teacher near you, call the American Association of Diabetes Educators toll-free at 1–800–TEAMUP4 (832–6874), or look on the Internet at *www. diabeteseducator.org* and click on "Find a Diabetes Educator."

Dietitians

To find a dietitian near you, contact the American Dietetic Association at *www.eatright.org* and click on "Find a Nutrition Professional."

Government

The National Heart, Lung, and Blood Institute (NHLBI) is part of the National Institutes of Health. To learn more about heart and blood vessel problems, write or call the NHLBI Health Information Center, P.O. Box 30105, Bethesda, MD 20824–0105, 301–592–8573; or see *www. nhlbi.nih.gov* on the Internet.

To get more information about taking care of diabetes, contact:

National Diabetes Information Clearinghouse

1 Information Way
Bethesda, MD 20892–3560
Phone: 1–800–860–8747
TTY: 1–866–569–1162
Fax: 703–738–4929
Email: ndic@info.niddk.nih.gov
Internet: www.diabetes.niddk.nih.gov

National Diabetes Education Program

1 Diabetes Way
Bethesda, MD 20814–9692
Phone: 1–888–693–NDEP (6337)
TTY: 1–866–569–1162
Fax: 703–738–4929
Email: ndep@mail.nih.gov
Internet: www.ndep.nih.gov

American Diabetes Association

1701 North Beauregard Street
Alexandria, VA 22311
Phone: 1–800–DIABETES (342–2383)
Internet: www.diabetes.org

Juvenile Diabetes Research Foundation International

120 Wall Street
New York, NY 10005–4001
Phone: 1–800–533–CURE (2873)
Internet: www.jdrf.org

Made in the USA
San Bernardino, CA
30 March 2014